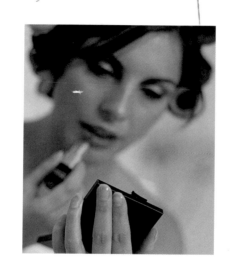

pocket
superflirt

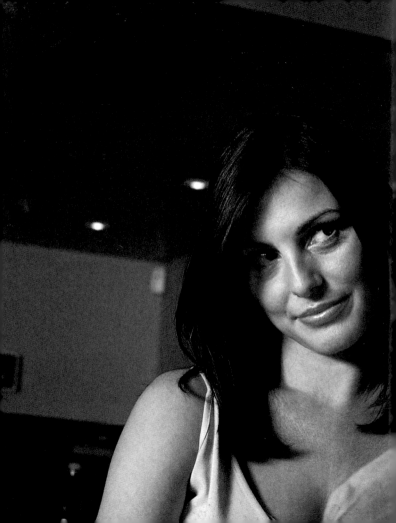

pocket superflirt

tracey cox

A Dorling Kindersley Book

LONDON, NEW YORK, MUNICH,
MELBOURNE, DELHI

Design XAB Design
Senior Editors Peter Jones, Dawn Bates
Art Editor Nicola Rodway
Managing Art Editor Emma Forge
Publishing Director Corinne Roberts
Art Director Carole Ash
DTP Designer Julian Dams

Photography by Janeanne Gilchrist at
Unit Photographic

First published in Great Britain in 2005
by Dorling Kindersley Limited,
80 Strand, London WC2R 0RL

A Penguin Company

2 4 6 8 10 9 7 5 3 1

Copyright © 2005 Dorling Kindersley Ltd.
Text copyright © 2005 Tracey Cox

This edition comprises extracts from
Superflirt © 2003 Dorling Kindersley Ltd.
Text copyright © 2003 Tracey Cox

A CIP catalogue record for this book is
available from the British Library.

ISBN 1 4053 0558 4

Reproduced by GRB, Italy
Printed and bound in Singapore
by Star Standard

See our complete catalogue at
www.dk.com

contents

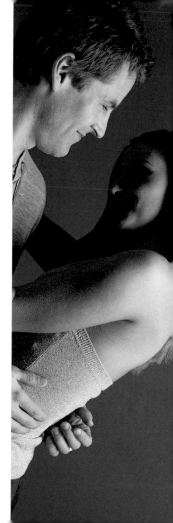

Introduction

Ever been out on a date and thought I wonder if they really fancy me or are just being polite? Ever watched someone watching you but both been too shy to make a move? Ever ended up home alone, kicking yourself for not having the courage to approach someone you liked? Slip *pocket superflirt* in your pocket or handbag next time you go out and this need never happen to you again! If you're searching for instant answers to these and other common dating dilemmas, this little book is your new must-have accessory.

> ## Want **on-the-spot answers** to all your **dating dilemmas?** This little book is your new **must-have accessory!**

Like the full-size version of *superflirt*, the main aim is to transform your love life. But the skills can also be used to improve your relationships with everyone from your workmates to your Mum. Packed with tricks, techniques and tips to make you irresistible to the opposite sex (or the same one, if that does it for you!), there are also oodles of revealing clues to help you sum someone up in a second. If you'd like to become a superflirt — a playful, warm, friendly, sizzlingly sexy creature — this book is for you!

Tracey X

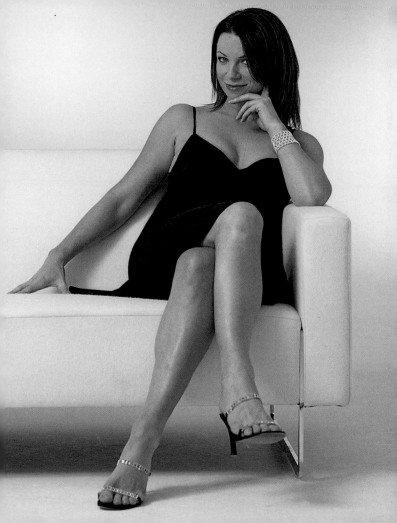

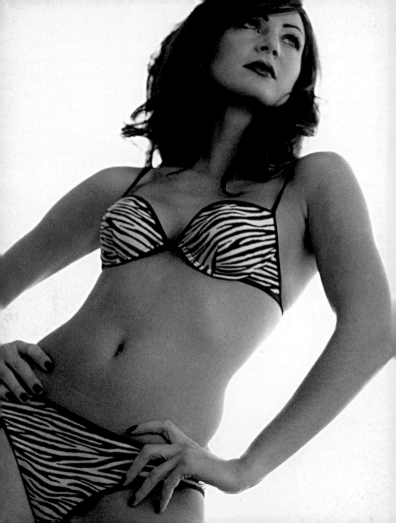

1 **Fake it!**

Alter your body language to look and feel instantly sexier and more confident.

Ask someone how humans communicate and it's likely they'll answer, "With words". The truth is, we signal around 12 things silently for every message delivered verbally. Almost all researchers agree 65 per cent of communication is through non-verbal body language – lots claim it's more like 90 per cent! Some of these body language signals we're conscious of making – giving a friend the thumbs up after they've made a great speech or winking at someone to share a private joke. Most, we're not. We all subconsciously send out a constant stream of other gestures that reveal our innermost thoughts and feelings. The way we walk, stand, sit, and hold ourselves reflects our perspective on life and how it's treated us. First impressions are hard to shake because they're often accurate – our body language reflects our personality in ways most of us aren't even aware of!

If you find all that a bit alarming, join the club. When I was first presented with this evidence, I too wanted to sit on my hands and not move a muscle ever again. Especially not in front of anyone I remotely fancied. Did this mean the guy sitting next to me at work could read my mind? Were my secret fantasies written all over my face? The answer is yes. If he knew enough about body language, he probably would be able to see through the ultra-cool façade to spot the true emotions (lust and infatuation) jostling just below the surface. Blimey! How embarrassing is that? Then something else occurred to me: if he can "read" what I'm really thinking, then I must be able to read him. And for anyone who's ever thought, "I wonder if they fancy me?" this is damn handy.

> # Positively **adjusting** your body language can drastically up **your chances** of someone liking, **loving,** or respecting you.

There's even more good news. Reading body language isn't just priceless when you're on the pull, interpreting your own body language can help you recognize hidden emotions. It also makes you aware of what signals you're sending others, helping you understand their reactions to you. Positively adjusting or actively altering your body language can drastically up your chances of someone liking, loving, or respecting you, often allowing you to get what you want without saying a word! How? Understanding body language allows you to gather information about people's feelings which they're too shy, polite, or uptight to admit or aren't even aware of themselves. An eyebrow flash (see p.52) lets you know someone fancies you before they've even registered the thought themselves. Fancy a flingette? Want a long-term partner? Want to make yourself generally more popular, confident, and authoritative? I can't think of a more effective way to do it than to master the art of body language.

A lot of what I'm going to talk about in this book relies on the "fake it till you make it" principle. This simply means if you alter your body language, you can alter your attitude, perceptions, and emotions. Yes, I know you want me to fast-forward to the eyebrow flash bit and skip the theory. I promise to do just that in a nanosecond, but to be really good at it, you first need to understand a few basics.

HOW IT CAN WORK FOR YOU

Because our body language reflects our personality, it follows that particular gestures and behaviours are associated with particular personalities. The simplest example is this: happy people smile, angry people frown. Put a smile on your face and people will assume you're happy, frown and they'll assume you're not. If you therefore imitate or adopt the body language gestures of the personality you'd like to have, you'll be seen as having that personality. Let's say you're shy. Act confident – stand up straight and look people in the eye – and people will think you're confident because that's how confident people behave. Now here's the magical part: because you're acting confident, people will now think you are. Never mind that inside you're a complete mess, all they see is a cool, confident exterior. This affects the way they react to you.

Confident people get asked for their opinions, so it's likely you will be too. While you're a bit nervous because this doesn't normally happen, you'll probably manage to volunteer something and – "Wow! I did it!" – suddenly feel a little bit important. You start to feel confident and the chain reaction continues. Initially you're faking it – pretending to be something your not. Do it long enough, and your body language will reflect the real you because you've become that person.

Don't get me wrong, I'm all for working on the cause not the symptom: you do need to address the issues that made you shy in the first place, as well as work on your body language. But whoever said there was an order to how we improve ourselves? We think too much sometimes. So how about you bypass the brain for a bit, forget about what you feel like on the inside and instead work on an outward illusion? Personally, I think it's more sensible. Change your body language and the mind often follows. Walk tall and your self-esteem lifts as well. Facial expressions are equally as mood-altering. It's called "the facial feedback effect": our expressions reinforce the emotion that caused them because the position of our facial muscles feeds information back to our brain. Stretch your mouth into a smile and the brain registers that we're smiling and releases the hormonal response that usually accompanies a real smile, feeling happy. Our "happy face" and "feeling happy" works backwards as well as forwards.

IT'S OKAY TO FAKE IT!

Hopefully, this goes some way to answering those who think it's being "false" to use body language or anything else that improves our external appearance because "it's what's inside that counts" and "it's bad or manipulative to pretend to be something you're not." Listen, I'm all for letting it all hang out once people get to know each other, but I vehemently believe, for certain situations like dates, job interviews, meeting the parents, it's in everyone's interest to present themselves in the best possible light. Most people make an effort to look good and be on best behaviour in those circumstances – particularly on a date. With good reason. What's underneath is important, but you've got to look OK and get the body language right for them to want to stick around and see what else you've got to offer.

Of course there will always be sceptics. Someone who says, "I crossed my arms just then because I was cold not defensive. See? I tricked you!" Not. You can't read someone based on one body language gesture – everyone has their own personalized body language. The idea is to look for clusters of gestures – lots of things pointing towards the same conclusion – rather than just one thing.

> What's **underneath is important**, but you've got to look OK for them to want to stick around and see **what else you've got to offer.**

It's not an infallible science and it certainly won't tell you everything – we need words as well. But it is an astonishingly perceptive and effective way to gather information. It could even help you predict the future of your relationship! Psychologist and relationships guru John Gottman studied 700 married couples over a long period. Part of his research involved videotaping the couples discussing stressful issues in their relationship or reminiscing about how they met. Afterwards, he analysed their body language, focusing on facial expressions (including real vs. fake smiles, curled upper lips, and rolling eyes). Based on what he learnt from this, Gottman was then able to predict with 75 per cent accuracy whether a couple would divorce within six years, simply by analysing three minutes of body language interaction on video. Give him 15 minutes and his accuracy score climbs to 85 per cent. Now that's impressive!

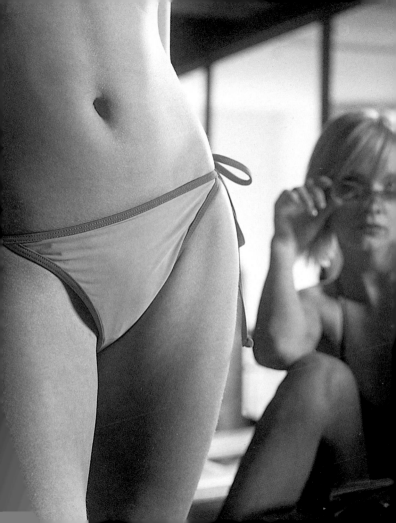

WALKING THE WALK

We all lead with a part of our body when we walk – it's the bit that looks as though it's being pulled forwards, ahead of everything else. Lead with your shoulders and you'll look protective and fearful. Lead with your knees and your legs look like they're carrying you places you don't want to go. If your chest enters the room before you do, you're at a risk of appearing pushy. The two best options for maximum effectiveness? A neutral walk – where no body part leads – or to lead with your pelvis. For the most dramatic results combine an exaggerated roll of the hips with squared shoulders, saucily swinging arms, direct eye contact and an ultra-confident facial expression.

- **Rolling hips** An exaggerated hip-swinging walk sends a powerful me-Jane, you-Tarzan sexual signal. Anatomical differences mean women have a greater rolling action of the pelvis. Switched-on females know rolling hips draw attention to hips, bum, and genitals and can mean the difference between attracting attention or being ignored.
- **Head held high** The higher our self-esteem, the higher we hold ourselves (actual height doesn't matter; it's presence and attitude that counts). A confident, raised head is a typical high-status display of a dominant individual.
- **Mirroring** Copying someone's walk is one of the quickest ways to glean clues of their true character. By imitating and getting "in step" with another person for mere minutes, you can understand their world and get a good taste of what it feels like to be them. Walk in a stressed person's shoes – fast, with purpose, looking straight ahead – and you'll start to feel anxious. Mirror an ambler and the anxiety dissolves into a hazy whatever-whenever horizon.

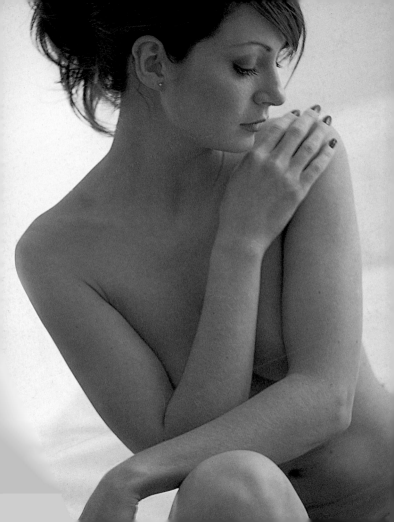

2 What if I'm shy?

Discover the five body language fix-its that will transform you from shy to casually confident in a mere 60 seconds. Instant assertiveness!

Before we get into specifics, I want to say something. Being shy isn't something to be embarrassed about. We're all shy in certain situations, some of us just cover it up better, that's all. I walked into a meeting two days ago with my tummy doing more backflips than an Olympic gymnast. I felt incredibly nervous and shy – but I didn't look it. And that's what this is all about: teaching you how to cover up shyness and getting you through the bit when the butterflies feel more like a colony of bats doing the can-can. It's the initial part that's the hardest – just about all of us eventually calm down and feel OK given a little time – so that's what we'll concentrate on here.

Why are some people shy and others not? It's usually got a lot to do with our upbringing. Confident parents breed confident kids simply because they expose their children to more people. If your home is overflowing with neighbours, friends, and family, you quickly learn the basic social skills of how to interact with strangers and make and keep friends without even trying. If you haven't had practice in the skills needed to turn an acquaintance into a friend, it's no wonder meeting strangers is daunting. The solution to beating shyness is to mount a two-fold campaign: work on raising low self-esteem (which tends to go hand in hand with shyness) and interact as much as possible with as many different people as possible. If you don't feel capable of doing this yourself, get help. There are lots of books, workshops, and counselling opportunities to help nudge you along a bit. While you're working on the inside, let me help by working on the outside and also giving you some practical advice on how to talk to strangers. Right! Now, let's go on to the five instant fix-its.

The first fix-it is to breathe   I know, you've heard this one before "Take a deep breath blah blah blah." Well, how about you do it? Because the first thing anyone does when they're feeling nervous or shy is to hold their breath. (The giveaway: taking very deep breaths occasionally, in an attempt to inject oxygen fast!) If you take a deep breath before speaking, it not only relaxes you, it gives you time to think. Another plus: it lowers the tone of your voice making you sound more authoritative.

Fix-it number two   Stand like a confident person: pull your tummy in, lift your chest to the ceiling, and square your shoulders by pulling them up to your ears, then back and down. Now, put your hands casually on your hips and make sure your body is directly facing the person you're talking to. This says "I'm giving you the best possible direct view of me because I'm happy with who I am and what I look like." (I know, inside you're cringing but this is all about externals, remember?) One final adjustment to the way you're standing: shift your weight so it's on one leg. A study of business executives showed per cent of high achievers will assume this pose – hands on hips, weight on one leg – within half an hour of you meeting them. Practise the pose in front of a mirror until it starts to look natural, then pay attention because fix-it three is the most important of the lot.

Fix-it number three The single, most effective way to change people's perception of you as shy, is to meet their eye. Easier said than done? Try this exercise: instead of looking at the pavement or downwards, look straight ahead. That's already a step in the right

> The single, **most effective way** to change people's perception of you as shy, is to **meet their eye.**

direction. From there, work up to glancing over to people's faces for a split second. Then, for a count of three, look at the tops of people's heads – you're not meeting their eyes, but looking vaguely at a point just above their forehead. The next step is to imagine their face is a circle and travel around it with your eyes. Then concentrate on their features – mouth first, nose next, then (finally) try focusing on their eyes. Depending on how shy you are, it might take anywhere from two days to a month of taking baby steps to work through this exercise and be able to look them in the eye, but persevere. There another great trick for the really, really shy which means you do ever have to make eye contact. Yes, really. When you're lookir at someone, instead of making eye contact, make nose cor Concentrate your gaze on the bridge of the person's nos of their eyes: very few people will notice the difference

Once you're able to meet people's eyes, practise making eye contact with as many people as possible – three strangers a day minimum. That's your target. When you're up to three people a day and you've done that for three days running, it's time to deliberately focus on people you find attractive. Now aim to make eye contact with three people you find attractive three times a week, then three times a day. Remember, you don't have to talk to them just yet so it's not too stressful. Just make eye contact and if you can possibly manage it, accompany that with a smile. That's more than enough to get you started and well on your way to the next part of our programme: chatting to strangers.

Fix-it number four   Make yourself look safe to talk to. I don't mean put down the machete and remove the hangman's mask, just look friendly, approachable, and happy in your skin. Make sure your body language is open. Uncross everything. Don't hunch your shoulders. Don't frown. Lift your head up. That's better. Now, get yourself into position…

Fix-it number five   If you don't naturally look confident, mimic those who do. By imitating their speech, style, and posture, you literally feel what it's like to walk through the world in their shoes, and you will appear more confident. This is a great way to unlock body language secrets, helping you adopt new confidence or new ways of communicating with people. When you find a you like, adopt it as your own. About the only things you mirror are negative body-language gestures or particularly they decide to stick a finger in their nose, ear, (or they're on their own.

HOW TO TAKE A COMPLIMENT

The first rule for taking a compliment: don't fish for one or you'll end up floundering. "So what's the best sex you've ever had?" I once asked an old boyfriend, settling back comfortably and waiting for the praise. He beamed. "Oh, without a doubt it was this Danish girl. She was *fan*-tastic." Get the point? (I certainly did). Besides, a compliment delivered after a prompt is a bit like someone saying "I love you" when you've just asked, "Do you love me?" It doesn't exactly make your heart or head swell does it? Never mind other bits.

> # **Compliments** aren't **ping-pong balls.**
> You don't have to **keep serving**
>   them back and forth, over and over.

There's only one thing you need to do if someone compliments you: smile and say thank you. Then simply continue with what you were doing or saying. People (women) find it difficult to do this for fear of looking vain. If we simply say "thank you", isn't that like agreeing with them? Won't they think we're – deep breath now – a bit too, well, happy with ourselves? This is why many women launch into that ridiculous "Oh, this old thing…" routine which does nothing except a) turn us into a cliché b) insinuate they've got bad taste. If you want to say something more, try "Thank you. That means a lot to me that you think that." Or, "Thank you. It's really nice of you to notice." Resist the urge to compliment them back. "You think I've got great hair, well, hullo! Yours is far nicer than mine." Compliments aren't ping-pong balls. You don't have to keep serving them back and forth.

HOW TO GIVE A COMPLIMENT

If the no-no for taking a compliment is don't ask for one, the don't-even-dream-of-going-there equivalent for giving a compliment is don't say it if you don't mean it. The second piece of advice: if you are going to give a compliment, make it as personal as possible. Ditch the "nice outfit" for "Your eyes look amazing against that grey top." Think of what you'd like to say, then substitute another word for the obvious. What's a better, more specific adjective than pretty/nice/smart/great? Also steer clear of the obvious body parts ("Gosh, you're tall!") and hone in on detail ("Haven't you got beautiful hands/lips/an infectious smile.") But most of all ask yourself: what is the person you're complimenting most proud of?

A compliment, said **behind our back** often means more than **one said to our face.**

Another great technique is "accidental adulation": slipping praise into an otherwise bland sentence. "This probably won't interest you but my sister's on this great diet…" (implication being you don't need to go on one). Passing on a compliment from someone else also works well. They're chuffed, they think more of the person who originally said it (a compliment said behind our back often means more than one said to our face), and you seem nice for passing it on. If you're too shy to compliment directly, this is a way of doing it: tell a mutual friend and let them repeat it. It makes you seem less sycophantic and is an effective way of letting them know they're admired.

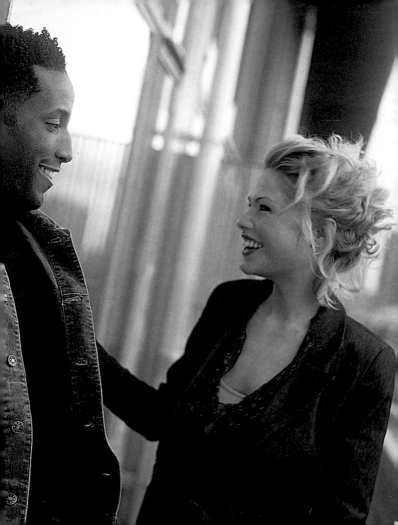

How to talk to strangers

MAKE CONTACT

Stand close enough to strike up a conversation but not so close they've got no choice. Catch their eye, smile briefly but brightly, wait for a second or two for a response, then look away. If they smile and make direct eye contact, they're open to talking. If they avoid your eyes and give a tight, closed-mouth smile, they're shy or not interested.

SAY SOMETHING

If there's one thing I want you to absorb from this chapter it's this: chat-up lines don't work. Rather than use a 'line', just say something appropriate to the situation you're in. If you're in a sandwich shop, saying, "Have you eaten here before? I can't decide between the chicken or the tuna" is going to work better than a corny chat-up line. The more ordinary the chat, the better.

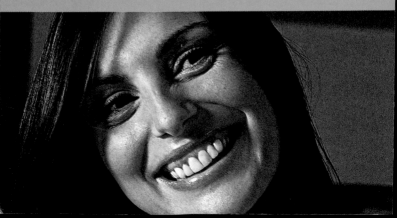

WHAT IF MY HEAD'S EMPTY?

The first lesson at journalism school is to answer five obvious questions in the first paragraphs of any story – who, what, when, where, and why. It's even more effective as a model for an opening line. Run through the five words and one's bound to inspire you.

KEEP IT GOING

Move from polite chit-chat to a real conversation by adding "feel" and "tell" questions. "Tell me why…" "How did you feel when…" Above all, keep smiling. Look like you're enjoying chatting to them and they'll be more likely to enjoy chatting to you.

ARE THEY WELL-MANNERED OR GENUINELY INTERESTED?

If someone's chatting out of politeness, they'll take the first chance they can to end the conversation. Test them out. Come up with a plausible excuse to leave their side for a few minutes and see if they're keen for you to come back.

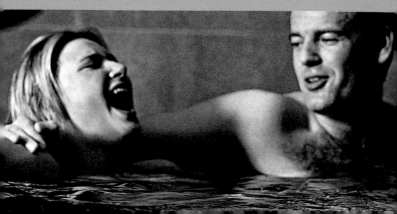

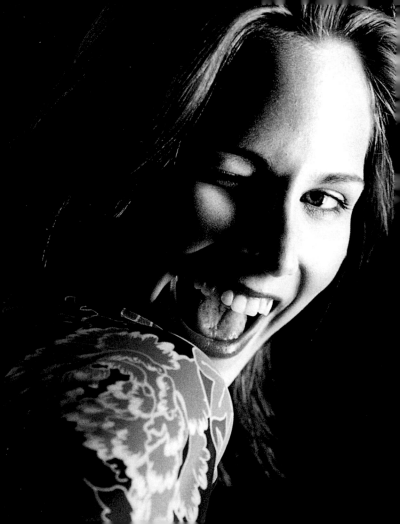

3 Optical illusions

From lowered lashes to wicked winks, eye contact is the ultimate flirting tool. Get this part right and the rest is easy.

A wink saved my life once. Well, my self-esteem anyway. It was the first time I'd returned to London after my parents emigrated to Australia and a friend of mine had put me in touch with a friend of his, who'd generously offered to let me stay. Christopher lived in Wimbledon and turned out to be incredibly posh. He was also funny, sexy, generous, and all-round fanciable. Which somehow made it even worse when he insisted on me joining him at a never-ending whirl of society functions. A 21-year-old student, my suitcase wasn't exactly bursting with Versace originals, so I was forced to turn up dressed in bizarrely inappropriate things. I remember standing awkwardly in a group at the Ascot races, convinced I was committing all sort of social sins (and was apparently), feeling gauche, unsophisticated, shy, and painfully out of place. (You try wearing Doc Martens and a mini-skirt surrounded by a sea of designer dresses). The only time I looked up was to steal a quick glance at Christopher, to see if he was as embarrassed at me being there as I felt. Rather than looking humiliated, he gave a sexy little smile and a big reassuring wink. In the blink of an eye, he'd said, "I know how you feel but you're doing fine. I'm here with you, relax." That wink was devastating. It made me feel accepted, sexy, admired, reassured, and downright bloody fantastic. It made me lift my head up, square my shoulders, meet the eyes of the person standing next to me and strike up conversation. In that moment, I went from having the worst time of my life to having the best time.

> It's virtually impossible to
> **connect and communicate** with
> someone without eye contact – let alone
> to **flirt or fall in love**.

In a tense situation that one small movement of the eye had a dramatic effect, and when you consider 80 per cent of our information about the outside world comes through our eyes, it's hardly surprising almost all dating experts rate eye contact as the ultimate flirting tool. It's virtually impossible to connect and communicate with someone without eye contact – let alone to flirt or fall in love. The real reason why superstars wear sunglasses at night isn't to look cool, it's to hide their emotions.

Eighteen times more sensitive than our ears, our eyes are capable of responding to one and a half million simultaneous messages. So finely tuned, they'll subconsciously spot when someone starts looking at us and start taking mental notes. If that person is checking everyone out, they'll stop registering the information; if it's just us they're interested in, they'll signal the brain to give us a nudge that someone's

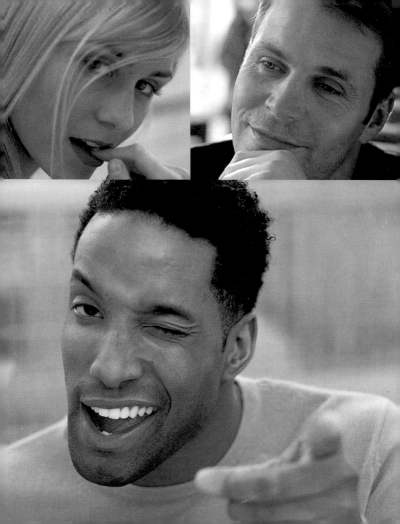

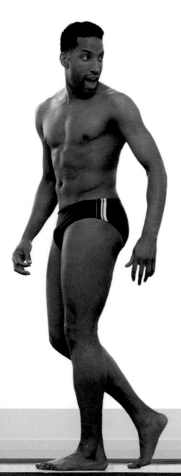

watching. (Forget the earth mother image. Mother Nature is a complete and utter sexpot!) Vital for communicating all emotions and particularly handy for interpreting sexual signals, it's hardly surprising this entire book is littered with references to eye-contact techniques. Here are just a few to get you started…

● **Focus attention** Draw attention to your eyes by using something to point to them. Our eyes automatically follow movement, so by pushing your hair away from your eyes or by tapping near them with a pen, you'll force anyone talking to you to look up and into your face. Another quick trick is to put your thumb underneath the side of your chin and rest your first and index fingers on the side of your face pointing towards your eyes. (An added bonus: not only will it draw attention to your eyes, it subliminally makes people think you're intelligent because you're pointing to your brain as well.)

- **The four-and-a-half second scan** A normal face scan lasts three seconds, scan for four and a half and it's clear they've "caught your eye". Eye contact of more than ten seconds between two people means one of two things: you're about to (or at least want to) fight or have sex. Prolonged eye contact produces intense emotional reactions regardless of whether it's a fist or a pair of lips heading your way. It activates the nervous system, raises our heart rate and blood flow, and stimulates the production of certain hormones. Just about everyone knows being watched is a sign that someone's interested, so the four-and-a-half second scan is a great way to subtly make your intentions known.

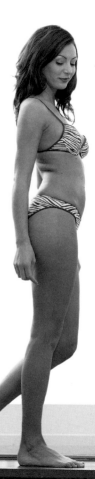

- **The slide and settle** Let your eyes settle on someone so they're aware you've noticed them, then as they're still watching you, slide your eyes around the room before settling back on them again. This effectively says, "You instantly attracted me and you're still the pick of the room even after I've checked out the competition." One other point while we're on the topic of eye slides – if you're interested, it's best to break the very first eye contact made by dropping your eyes straight down, then directly up again to lock eyes after a few seconds. If someone's eyes instead slide away from yours to the side or upwards and don't return after a minute or two, they're almost definitely not interested. The slide and settle is a quick movement – the whole thing's over in 10–15 seconds – but it's impressively accurate.

- **The flirting triangle** Eye movement studies show we look at different parts of other people's faces depending on the situation and level of attractiveness. When looking at strangers or in business situations, we make a small triangle by moving our eyes from eye to eye, dipping them as we move across the bridge of the nose. With friends or in more friendly social situations, the triangle widens as our eyes drop below eye level to include the nose and the mouth. With lovers and people we fancy, the triangle broadens even further, dropping below the mouth to include the breasts and other good bits like the genitals. The more intense the flirting, the more concentrated the eye contact becomes at certain parts of the triangle. When we're in full flirting mode, eye to eye contact becomes fast, furious and constant, seconded by long periods spent staring at the mouth. Our eyes spend the rest of the time making little side journeys to the bits at the bottom of the triangle.

- **Blink if you fancy them** It's easy to see where the term "batting your eyelashes" originated from: if someone looks at us and likes what they see, they tend to blink more. Because the brain associates rapid blinking with finding someone sexually attractive, the more you blink at someone, the more attracted you feel to them. This, of course, can be manipulated for your benefit! You can increase the blink rate of the person you're talking to, by simply blinking more yourself. If the person likes you, they'll unconsciously try to match their blink rate to keep in sync

A quiet **wink matched with a sexy smile** can be incredibly bonding simply because it's secret and implies the two of you are **closer than others present.**

with you, which in turn, makes you both feel more attracted to each other! Don't assume slow blinking means disinterest however. If we're completely absorbed in a task or addictively entertained, we blink very little. Confused? Don't be. Common sense and other body language signals will tell you which interpretation applies to your situation.

- **...and wink if you want more** As evidenced by my little story, a quiet wink matched with a sexy smile can be incredibly bonding simply because it's secret and implies the two of you are closer than others present.

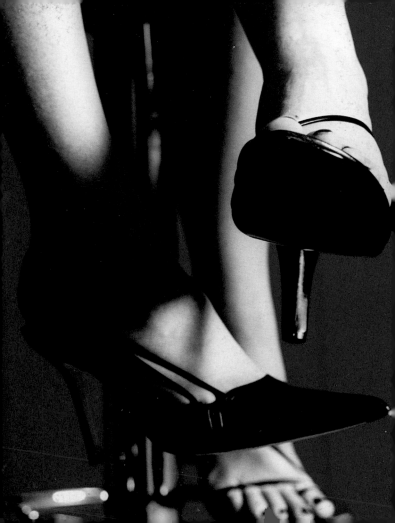

Flirty footwork

Legs give away loads about our true intentions and all of us find ourselves flirting with our feet.

There's a friend of mine who I fancy like mad and he does me. We confessed after a billion bottles of wine one night but for a billion boring and complicated reasons, neither of us is prepared to act. While our heads accept the logic, and mentally we've moved on, our bodies refuse point-blank to give up. Take the other night. We plonked ourselves in separate armchairs and settled in to watch a video, both facing forwards in typical telly-watching mode. Totally engrossed, our bodies rearranged themselves without our permission. The credits rolled and we looked down to see ourselves practically climbing out of our seats towards each other. Arms dangled over the edge of our chairs, our bodies had turned away from the screen and towards each other, one leg stretched forwards and our ankles intertwined. "Blimey," we said. "And that's without a drink!"

We put on the face we want others to see but our body language reveals our true feelings. Hands are halfway down and we're semi-conscious that they're liable to "leak" secret emotions. Legs and feet, however, tend to be left to their own devices – which is why they're so remarkable for giving clues about what's really going on.

THEY'RE KEEN IF:

- **Their feet point towards you** If they're standing, one leg will move a step in your direction.
- **Their legs are crossed and the top leg points towards you** The direction of the leg cross is important. If you're sitting side by side and they cross towards you, you're on friendly turf.

If they **stroke your foot** with their toes and you still **don't budge** or you reciprocate, it's effectively saying, **"I will go home with you."**

- **They're sitting with legs wide apart and feet firmly planted on the floor, directly facing you** This person is confrontational, secure, sexual, and effectively saying, "Here I am. Take a good look at what's about to be yours." If they're leaning forwards and fixing you with a steady gaze, there's good reason why you feel like a lamb before the slaughter. They're moving in for the kill.
- **Playing footsie** People tend to use this technique when it would be embarrassing to be seen obviously flirting with someone, like a group of colleagues on a night out or at a dinner party where everyone's married. It works like this: they put their foot next to yours so it's touching. You don't move. They snuggle their foot in closer so you know it's not a mistake, you apply slight pressure back. If they risk stroking your foot with their toes and you still don't budge or you reciprocate, it's effectively saying, "I will go home with you."

If you're a guy reading this you're in luck. You get extra info because women use their legs to send more flirting signals than men. Why? Think about it, men's bits get in the way!

SHE'S KEEN IF:

- **She's crossed her legs at the thighs** The classic "I fancy you" female flirting signal. So clichéd, it's potent – everyone can read it, everyone responds to it.

- **The double twist** If she twines one leg around so her foot crosses behind her calf and also the ankle, you're even more in luck. Hinting at creativity (it's a little more imaginative than a normal leg cross), flexibility (always handy), and all the tension of a coiled spring (if she's physically wound herself in a knot, it must mean pent up sexual frustration – which you, of course, will be happy to relieve.) Favoured by tall women with gazelle-length limbs (it works better with long legs than short), this pose is often paired with a little-girl gesture -- like a finger, seductively twirling hair – to downplay any possible height superiority.

- **She keeps on crossing and uncrossing her legs** The more deliberately it's done, the more interested she is. It's a not-so-subtle ploy to draw attention to the legs and genital area.

- **She's kicking one leg up and down, while crossed, or dangling a shoe from her toes** This girl's up for more than just coffee. It's a thrusting motion designed to mimic more intimate thrusting. Gulp.

- **She slips her foot slightly out of her shoe** She's incredibly comfortable with you and the situation. If you want to test her reaction to something, do it now. If she feels ill at ease, that shoe will be shoved back on very quickly.

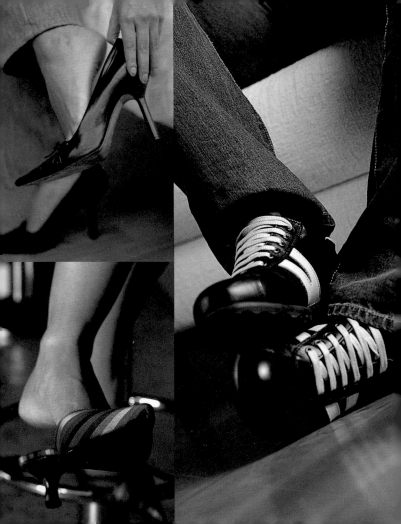

NOT SO GREAT FOR EITHER SEX…

- **Their legs are crossed but your instinct tells you all is not well** The standard leg cross – right leg rested over left – is usually a sign someone is relaxed but it can also be a subtle way of protecting and forming a barrier. This is where it all gets a bit tricky. There's crossing legs in a sexy way to say "Check them – and me – out", and there's crossing legs to say "Stop looking at them and me." After all, keeping the upper thighs pressed together hides our most vulnerable area – the crotch. If they've also folded their arms, turned their head away, and averted their eyes, it's not good news. If they've recently plonked a bag or cushion on their lap, even worse. The ultimate "bugger off", would be for them to lean forwards and away from you, lifting a shoulder to effectively form a third barrier. (At this point, just slink away.)

- **They do the opposite to what you do** If they seem intent on adopting a different leg position to you, they're showing dominance or trying to emphasize how unlike you both are. ("See? We even sit differently.") Not a particularly welcome sign if you're so keen, you're practically panting.

- **They're rising up and down on their heels, swaying from side to side (sober), tapping their feet, shifting weight from foot to foot, or doing any sort of leg or feet jiggling** All point to a secret desire to walk or run away. This could be prompted by fear (they like you but you frighten the hell out of them) or disinterest. They might pretend to be fascinated and/or totally at ease but their feet are trying every possible way to get them out of there by trying to run without moving. Ease up on the flirting, make general soothing chit-chat, and see if it stops. If it does, it's safe to assume they were nervous and/or feeling intimidated. Didn't work? Sorry but it probably does mean you're not their cup of tea! Gather the few tatters of dignity you have left, wrap them around your shoulders, give a theatrical yawn, and tell them as much as you're enjoying yourself, you really must go home.

- **Their legs are tightly crossed** The tighter the cross, the more defensive the mood. If you're chatting to a woman and she lifts one leg, bends it at the knee, and wraps her hands around it, hugging it to her, back off. This is a classic protect-the-genitals position. Watch young girls forced to be nice to men they perceive to be "creepy" and they'll adopt this position involuntarily.

> If they're sitting with **knees together** and feet flat on the floor they're *not* someone to throw around **the bedroom.**
> Moving right along then...

- **They've crossed their legs and one foot is flapping up and down** They're tense and anxious and want to "get it over with" or are impatient to "get on with it". Judge quickly and act immediately. If you're in heavy flirting mode, it's a female doing it to you, and it's a bigger, more noticeable, faster movement, this is a VERY GOOD SIGN. She's impatient for things to progress NOW. Grab the moment or you might just lose it (and her). If all other signs hint at boredom, they're trying to amuse themselves until you finish that l-o-n-g story about the knee operation you had when you were 12. Sometimes the kicking is so aggressive, it's as though they want to kick the person who is boring them.

PICK A PERSONALITY FROM THE WAY SOMEONE SITS

- **Knees together, legs side by side, feet flat on the floor and neatly in line** The school prefect. On time, tidy, well-groomed, meticulous, not someone to throw around the bedroom. (Moving right along then…)

- **Knees together, toes together, heels apart** Shy and nervous. Coax them out of their shell as you'd lure a timid kitten down from a tree.

- **Legs crossed at the knees, top leg slightly kicking up and down** Cool, scheming, thoughtful, ambitious. I suspect they've got their eyes narrowed as they sweep them your way.

- **Legs stretched out, one foot resting on the other** The ultimate relaxed leg pose. They're at home, confident, and self-assured. Study the circumstances they're adopting the pose in, and you've got a strong clue of what makes them tick.

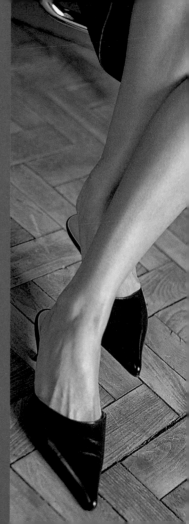

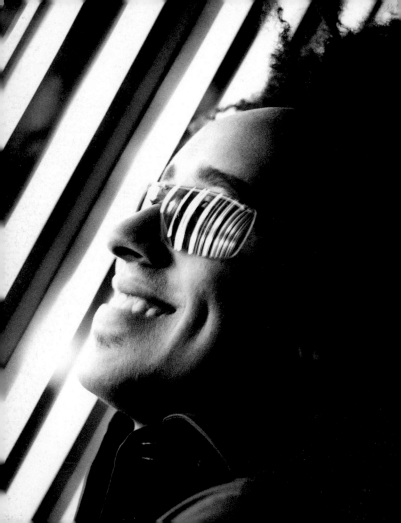

5 Babe magnet

Here's where you learn some sneaky, simple, and oh-so-effective ways to mesmerize her from your very first meeting.

Pocket Superflirt is crammed with tips and hints on how to make yourself more attractive to women. Just in case you're not entirely satisfied, however, here are a few more.

ON THE PULL

- **Look for "shiny" eyes** If she's gazing up at you with twinkly eyes that seem to sparkle with excitement, it's highly likely that she's interested in you. Chances are you've aroused her emotions – with a bit of luck, something like passion or adoration. The way it works is this: intense feeling causes the tear glands to secrete fluid but if the emotions aren't intense enough to produce tears and an overflow, the liquid pools instead. Excess moisture causes light to bounce more easily off the eyeball, making the eyes "dance" and look more attractive. This response can't be faked either, so glistening eyes are a good indicator you're having an effect on her. Be warned though, fear, stress, and discomfort manifest in exactly the same way so, as always, look for other signs that she fancies you.

- **Take a visual voyage** It doesn't matter how much of a good sort you are, if someone locks eyes with us for too long at a time, most of us feel like a butterfly with its wings pinned. Thing is, it's rather easy to become mesmerized when you're gazing at someone who's so damn sexy, you're practically dribbling. Fix it by forcing yourself to feast on the entire spread laid in front of you – in other words, take a visual voyage. As you're chatting to her, take time to check out her cute nose, the curve of her cheek, neck, and shoulders. Hover around her hairline, look at her earlobes, caress her entire face with your eyes. The trick to making your target feel admired rather than minutely examined is to make sure you keep the visual voyages short – flick back to her eyes for long seconds in between. Later, when all systems are go and you're ready to move it forwards into a kiss, it's OK – and even desirable – to make it obvious you're studying every part of her. On the topic of staring though…

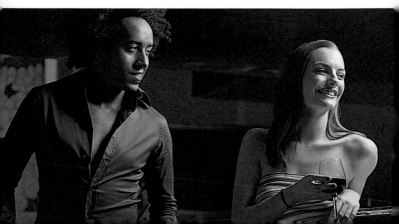

- **Gaze, don't stare** Initially, a flirty "I think you're a bit of alright" look should only last the time it takes you to say it out loud. In the beginning, you're playing a game of "I see you, do you see me too?", using your eyes to signal a quick expression of interest. (It's only later that longer periods of eye contact come into play.) Pay attention here guys because this is when it can all go horribly wrong. Stares can easily be mistaken for glares and there's a crucial difference between gazing and staring. When we gaze, our face is softer. Dreamy eyes, a half smile, and slightly lowered eyelids all indicate we're floating off into daydreams about the person we're looking at. A stare is much harder: a set, stern mouth, lips pressed together, wide, unblinking eyes, and an unwavering expression all mean you're curious or fascinated by what you're looking at…but not necessarily in a good way. The thing is, what feels like a gaze from your end can look like a stare/glare from theirs because of our individual mannerisms and

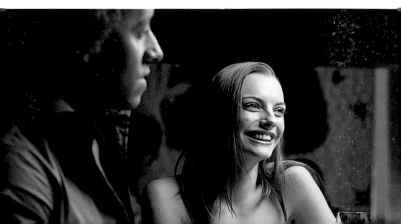

face shapes. If you're worried your come-on look is killing your chances, grab a mirror and see for yourself. If your gaze seems too hard, imagine you're looking at the person you adore most in the world and watch your eyes and face instantly soften, open, and relax. Restrict your gazes to no longer than five-second bursts until you're almost at kissing stage…then feel free to lock eyes (and limbs) for as long as you like.

● **Test they're flirting with you** If you're pretty sure they fancy you, up the stakes by very obviously making a play. Whisper something in their ear and let your lips touch their cheek as you're doing it, pull back, and make gooey eyes. Use every trick in the book to make it obvious you think they're sex on legs. If they're interested, they'll mirror you by increasing the intensity of their flirting. If they're not – or they're flirting without intent (having fun but don't plan on taking it further) – they'll tone down their

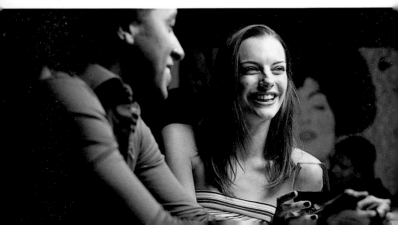

advances or stop flirting. You made it clear it was crunch-time – make a move or move on – and they've responded.

ON A DATE

- **Value yourself** You know what it's like: you open a birthday present and instantly think "Yuk!" You'd asked for a new wallet and that you got, but this one looks decidedly tacky. Shiny leather, childish stitching, a garish colour – it's got "return me" written all over it. "I hope you like it because it cost a fortune," beams the giver, "It's a designer label. [Insert name of famous popstar] has one apparently…" Before your very eyes, the wallet transforms: the shine suddenly oozes street cred, childish becomes artistic, and what was going straight back to the shop suddenly goes straight into your pocket. It's called perception: if we perceive something as expensive, it becomes valuable. Do your own designer branding by placing a value on your own worth: in

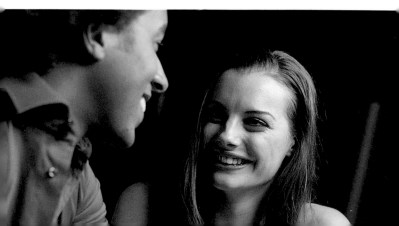

other words, act like you're worth a billion and she'll see you that way as well. I'm not talking about pretending you're wealthy or acting like you're way out of her league. I'm talking about behaving as though you're well and truly worthy of her affection. Which you are. The trick to pulling it off? Be attentive but not 24/7 available; pay compliments but keep her guessing.

> # Lay on the lines **too fast, too thick,** too early, and they'll all seem meaningless. Later, **she'll kill to hear them**.

That all sounds complicated, but it's dead easy if you follow one simple rule: don't shut out the rest of your life just because she's in it. That way, your friends/work/life will naturally intrude on your time and you won't be there to return every phonecall seconds after she's called or see her every time she clicks her fingers. The second bit of sneakery: load on the '"I think you're great" flattery without telling her how much you seriously like her. In other words, keep it as a general compliment ("You've got such a great smile"), rather than a protestation of love ("Every time you smile my heart flip-flops"). Lay on the lines too fast, too thick, too early, and they'll all seem meaningless. Later, she'll kill to hear them.

● **Track her down** Calling up to say, "How did that meeting go?" rather than the usual "How are you?" will put you light-years ahead of the competition. If you can't remember half the stuff she rattles on about, take notes. Seriously. Write things like "Ask if Sarah's sister had baby" and "S goes to doctor today" in your diary. Refer to it. If you're dead keen this should come naturally but sometimes the opposite happens – you're so nervous about getting everything else right, you forget the obvious. It's called tracking and it shows you've been listening and you care.

A FEW DATES LATER AND YOU'RE...
...ON A ROLL

- **Avoid an argument** You've had a few great dates and now this! As far as you're concerned, it's crystal clear you're right and she's wrong. Sadly, she's behaving as though you're talking in tongues (and not the sort she usually likes) and can't seem to get your point at all. If this happens to you, do something (anything) to get her moving. The quickest way to budge a mind lock is to get someone to change their body position. If she's sitting down, invent a reason for her to get up and walk around the room. If she's standing, get her to sit down. When our body is in a fixed position, our mind becomes frozen as well. There's no easier way to snap someone out of something than to get them to move.

- **Capture the moment** The opposite is also true. If you're locked together in a moment so intimate, you're afraid to breathe lest you ruin it, you're wise to grit your teeth and hang on (no matter how desperate the urge to pee). Get the timing wrong by "abandoning" her – lean back, leave to go to the bathroom, attract the attention of the waitress for another drink – and you may well lose the opportunity to move the relationship onto a deeper and more intense level.

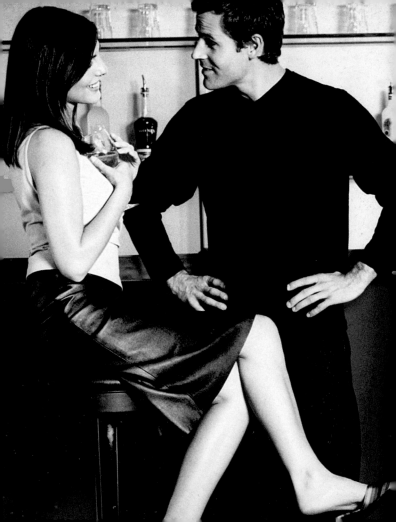

6 Is he interested?

You may think he's playing it cool, but take a closer look to discover the dozens of tell-tale signs that reveal his true feelings.

Legend has it men make the first move, then plead, cajole, wine, dine, and basically bribe (via chocolates, flowers, and dinner dates) women into their bachelor pads to either a) have their wicked way or b) get down on bended knee. Women – sweet, passive, delicate little flowers that we are – start out strongly by defying his attentions, until sheer persistence breaks down our resistance and we agree to…a sherry. Meanwhile, we fill our days by reading romance novels and twitching the net curtains, on the watch for knights on white stallions.

What a load of bollocks. Women have always made the first move and orchestrated the pace, flow, and direction of romantic relationships. Masters of intuition and emotional manipulation, women are adept at body language, able to gauge the emotional temperature of a room quicker than our nipples stiffen in a breeze. You can bet your next G&T, if he's on his way over, armed with courage and a chat-up line, you were the one who lured him there. Women choose from no less than 52 moves to show men they're interested. The average bloke chooses from a maximum of 10 to attract a female. In case you're not as good as the average female at deciphering body language, I've included the obvious along with more subtle, secretive, and (occasionally) downright loony signals.

IT'S ALL GOOD NEWS

- **He'll serve you an eyebrow flash** When we first see someone we're attracted to, our eyebrows rise and fall. If they fancy us back, they raise their eyebrows. This lasts about a fifth of a second and happens to everyone, regardless of age, race, or class. Lifting our brows pulls the eyes open and allows more light to reflect off the surface, making them look bright, large, and inviting. A flash might be easy to miss but they're so reliable, if you do spot one, you may know someone fancies you before they know it themselves. Deliberately extend it for up to one second and you've drastically upped the chances of him getting the message you're interested.

- **His face "opens"** If he likes what he sees, his lips will automatically part for a moment when your eyes first lock, and his nostrils will flare. Along with the raised brows and wide eyes this gives his face a friendly "open" expression.

- **He'll try to attract your attention** Some men might simply make a subtle tie adjustment. Others turn into Beppe the Clown and become so loud and boisterous, they're practically juggling and doing handstands. Any exaggerated movement or gesture usually means he's trying to stand out from the group. Another giveaway: he'll unconsciously detach from his friends by standing slightly apart, hoping to be seen as an individual.

- **He'll stroke his tie or smooth a lapel** We all know what these preening gestures mean. They're the equivalent of the female lip lick – "I want to look good for you."

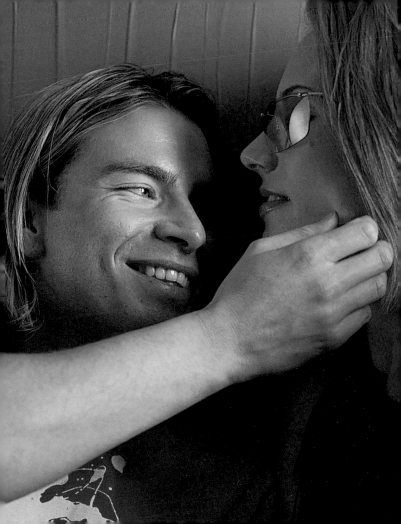

- **He'll smooth or muss up his hair**. Guys do this involuntarily and more often than you think. Glance back and look at him next time you trot off to the loo and I bet his hands are already on their way to touch his head.
- **His eyebrows remain slightly raised while you're talking** A slightly surprised, quizzical expression means he finds you fascinating. Or completely bonkers. Quite frankly, either are preferable to a man who looks at you with a smooth, relaxed brow and eyes. That one simply finds you boring.
- **He'll fiddle with his socks and pull them up** In the old days, men only dressed up on special occasions and while the suit might have survived months in mothballs, the socks invariably continued to get worn (to death). That's why he spent half the night pulling them up, in an attempt to look the part. It's an extension of preening and it's astonishingly accurate. If a guy pulls up or adjusts his socks in your presence, it's an almost 100 per cent sign he's interested and trying to look his best.

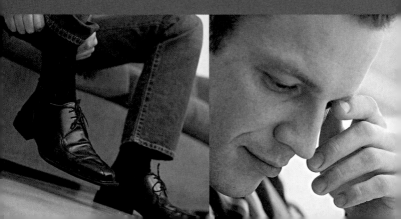

SECRET SIGNALS HE'S UP FOR IT...

- **Everything is erect** Ahem. What I mean is he'll stand with all his muscles pulled tight, to show his body off. He'll also stand directly in front of you to show full attention and lean forwards.

- **He'll let you see him checking out your body** He scanned your body automatically the second he laid is eyes on you. The difference here is you see him do it. The message: I'm considering you as a sexual partner.

- **He'll spread his legs while sitting opposite, to give you a crotch display** He's letting you have a good look at what's on offer. Hopefully he still has his jeans or trousers on at the time.

- **He'll stand with his hands on his hips** This accentuates his physical size and suggests body confidence. It's also a pointing gesture. We point with our hands at our best sexual assets and at the parts of our body we'd most like to be touched. If he has his hands on his hips, fingers splayed and pointing downwards, he's willing you to look, touch, and admire the bit he's proudest of.

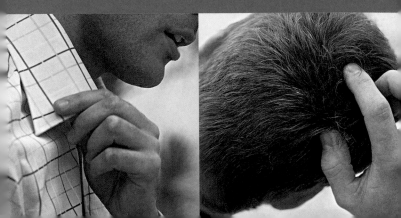

- **He'll play with the buttons on his jacket** This shows you've made him a little nervous plus he has an unconscious desire to remove his clothes. The next stage is to push the jacket open and hold it there by putting his hands on his hips. If he takes it off completely, he's imagining his shoes under your bed.

- **He'll touch his face a lot, while looking at you** He'll stroke his cheek with the back of his fingers, touch his ears, or rub his chin. When we're attracted to someone, our skin (most noticeably our lips and mouth) become increasingly sensitive to touch and other stimulation. If you smoke, you'll take more drags on your cigarette. If you're drinking, you'll take more sips. You start touching your own mouth more because your lips are ultra-sensitive and it feels good. Plus it plants the idea in the other person's mind that it could be a good idea to kiss you…

- **He'll start squeezing his glass or can or roll it from side to side, slightly squeezing it as he does so** When men are sexually interested, they start playing with circular objects. Why? They remind him of your breasts: his body is "leaking" what's happening in his subconscious mind.

- **He'll perch on the edge of his seat to get closer** And if he crosses his legs, the top leg will point in your direction.

- **He'll guide you by putting his arm on your elbow or in the small of your back** He's making sure he knows exactly where you're going by taking you there. It also shows you're being "taken care of" so no other men need volunteer.

- **He'll lend you his coat or jumper** This is a protective, sexy, ownership gesture. It says "what's mine is yours", something that's been close to their skin is now close to yours. Plus, it links you: he has to hang around to get it back.

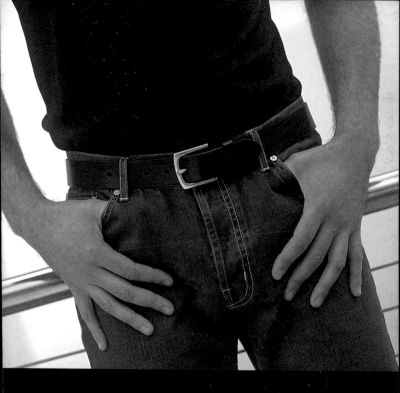

If he has his **hands on his hips**,
fingers splayed and pointing downwards,
he's willing you to look, touch and
admire **the bit he's proudest of**.

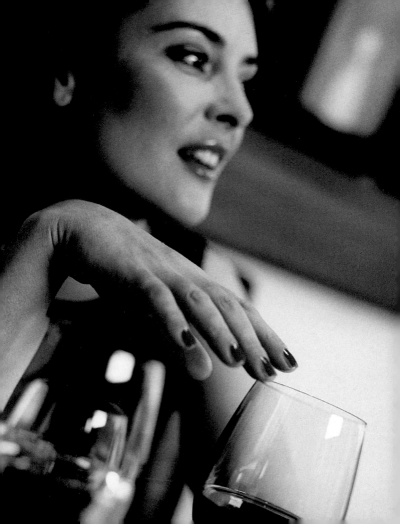

7 Is she interested?

> She may not "chat you up", but look out for the numerous non-verbal signals that show she definitely wants to get to know you more.

Interpreting female body language isn't as difficult as you think. It's firmly rooted in logic. Just about all flirtatious behaviour aims to accomplish one of three things: get us noticed by the person we fancy, get us closer to them, and get them to have sex with us. (I thought you'd like the last one, even if the reason is procreation rather than recreation.) When we're attracted to someone, our subconscious gives in to a natural urge to get close to that person. Mother Nature, thinks, "Here's a prospective population booster" and rings "all systems go!" alarm bells, instructing the rest of the body to look its best. She also connects with primitive, basic mating urges, suggesting they waft out some strong pheromone scents, and put the body on sexual standby. (Is it any wonder we're all obsessed with sex?)

Understand the theory and you'll start to see that most body language gestures make perfect sense. (When I meet someone delicious – or simply feel like a bit – I find myself stroking my lower tummy. Not only is this site fertility headquarters, it also happens to be the place most females first register a pang of desire.)

If you're an intelligent bloke, you've probably already figured out women initiate contact around two-thirds of the time. Rather than going up and chatting, however, they do it by giving you the green light to approach them, via non-verbal flirting signals. This is the sole reason why most men think they've make the first move – they're usually the ones who swagger over to speak. While it might not be the first move, it is possibly the bravest. Crossing the floor isn't easy and few women risk it. Reduce your chances of face-to-face humiliation by becoming a master at reading the sexual signals that drew you there. These will give you a massive head start…

IT'S ALL GOOD NEWS

● **She's looking at your mouth loads** It starts with the flirting triangle and becomes more intense as the flirting intensifies. The more infatuated she is, the more time she'll spend looking at your mouth while you're talking. If you've been doing a bit of autoerotic touching, she's got the hint and is fixated on it, imagining what it

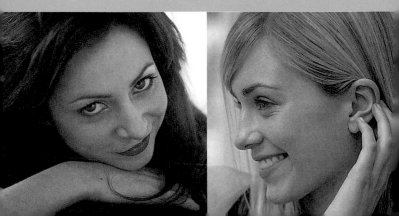

would be like to have your mouth on hers. Lick your lips and you'll see her focus shift to your tongue. Gosh! I wonder what she's thinking about now?

- **She's lightly stroking her outer thigh** We stroke ourselves for two reasons: to draw attention to a body part (eyes tend to follow fingers) and to subconsciously tease the person watching (bet you wish you were doing this).

- **She's checking out your bum** Both sexes scan the body of a potential mate but do it very differently. Being more visual and usually more sexually aggressive, men scan from the ground up, eyes sliding over feet, legs, crotch, tummy, breasts, shoulders, and (finally) the face. Women scan less obviously and in a different order. They start at the face, having a good look at the eyes and mouth, then move on to hair and overall size and build. His clothes and accessories (a wedding ring, watch, shoes) are next, finishing on his legs and then back up to check out his crotch and…his bottom. It's a long journey from your eyes to your ass

She'll lick her lips, fluff her hair, and **generally preen** while looking at you. "I'm making myself look even more attractive – **and it's all for you."**

and the fact she's got that far means you probably passed on the other counts. If you've been chatting for a while, glance backwards next time you leave her for drinks/the loo. If her eyes zoom downwards, she thinks you're sexy. (If she's looking horrified, all those pizzas in front of the telly have taken their toll.)

- **Her shoulders flash** When we meet someone we like we don't just flash our eyebrows for a split second, we also do a shoulder flash. Without realizing it, we'll shrug our shoulders when we meet someone we find attractive. It's a small, quick movement but stay alert to it if you want to be one step ahead of the game.

- **She lets a strap fall off a shoulder** Revealing a shoulder is incredibly provocative. So is a glance back over one or stroking her own. Even shrugging your shoulders can be sexy if it's done in the right way.

- **She starts massaging her neck** Didn't I tell you women are great at this manipulation stuff? She doesn't really have a stiff neck, she's just aware this pose lifts her breasts and exposes her armpit (another sexual hotspot).

- **She'll stand with her legs apart, weight on one foot and hips tilted** This is the stance of a high achiever: researchers studied executives at seminars and found 75 per cent assumed this position within half an hour. It's also the posture of a sexually supremely confident woman.

- **She'll dart short, repetitive glances your way** This says "Of all the things I could look at, you're the most interesting to me."

- **She looks straight at you and flips or tosses her hair** Some women toss, flicking their hair back with a head movement, others flick it back, using their hand. The second isn't just preening: by lifting her arm and brushing it through her hair, she's wafting pheromones in your direction from the sweat glands of her underarm (I know, far too much information). If she catches your attention, does either a toss or a flick, then looks back again, get yourself over there.

- **She'll flash her wrists** Wrists are a definite erogenous zone. Back in the days when women wore neck to knee clothing, the wrist and ankles were the only flesh ever exposed in public. Watch groups of women smoking to see a dramatic illustration of wrist turning as a flirting tool. Surrounded by just her girlfriends, each girl will usually have her wrist turned to face her own body whenever she lifts her cigarette to her mouth. The second a gorgeous guy appears, all wrists, magically and in unison, tend to turn outwards or to the side.

- **She'll lick her lips, fluff her hair, and generally preen while looking at you** "I'm making myself look even more attractive – and it's all for you."

- **Her hands start to glide over her arms and neck** Yep – it's autoerotic touching at work again.

- **She'll do a whisper and lean** If she lowers her voice and moves her head close to yours, she's inviting you to share her personal space. It's a thinly disguised ploy – if she speaks so quietly, you're almost obliged to lean forwards – but it works every time.

- **She moves her head closer to yours generally** The more we desire someone, the closer our heads get. The effect is two-fold: it excludes anything else from our field of vision and unconsciously prepares us for the first kiss. The most intimate pre-kiss position possible is where both your eyes are in line with each other's but still clearly in focus.

- **She'll sit with her inner thigh exposed** If one leg's tucked under her, revealing her inner thigh, and her head and body also point towards you, consider yourself wanted. She's revealing quite an intimate part of her body you'd normally only see during sex.

> **A huge genuine smile** delivered with direct eye contact is still the clearest signal of all **she wants you** to come over and talk to her.

- **She smiles broadly** A huge, genuine smile delivered with direct eye contact is still the clearest signal of all she wants you to come over and talk to her.
- **She'll fidget with her clothes** When we're aroused by someone, our clothes seem suddenly restrictive. Lots of people start removing layers, undo buttons, or hike up skirts. Note how many buttons she's got undone and see if a few more have magically freed themselves while you were getting drinks. Keep an eye on her thighs as well (I know, it's a hard job) to see if her hemline has risen along with your expectations.
- **She'll start invading your space with objects** Unfortunately, it's more likely to be a wine glass, rather than the keys to her apartment or personal body parts. If you're in a restaurant or bar, she'll gradually push her wine glass from her side of the table over to yours. If she's confident you're attracted to her, she'll leave it (and her hands) there, hoping you'll touch them.

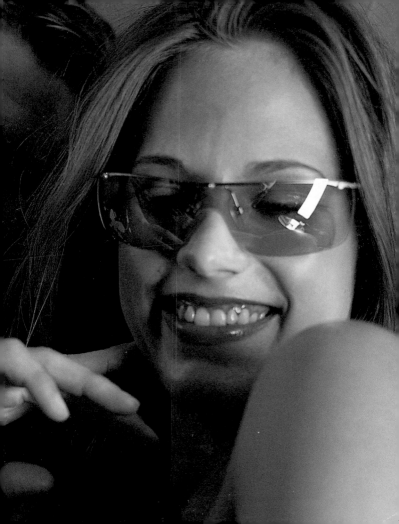

8 Falling in love

Absolutely crazy about someone? Discover the scientific spells and potent potions that will up your chances of making them fall for you.

Sometimes you can spend six months living, breathing, dripping, drooling, loving, and lusting after someone with zero result. And it's when that happens that the techniques which follow suddenly seem like a gift from heaven. Besides, it's not like I'm proposing black magic or suggesting any of these techniques will force someone to fall in love with you against their will. (If they did, I'd currently be shacked up with Brad Pitt.) What they will do though is nudge the odds a lot higher in your favour. Is that really so bad? I don't think so. Go on, keep reading. You know you want to…

HANG AROUND LOTS…BUT THEN BE UNAVAILABLE
The more you interact with someone, the more they'll like you, says David Lieberman, a US expert in human behaviour. He's right, actually. Several studies show repeated exposure to practically any stimulus makes us like it more (the only time it doesn't hold true is if our initial reaction to it is negative). So forget about being all aloof, evasive, and unavailable in the beginning. Instead, find loads of excuses to spend time with them.

Now, pay attention because this is the tricky bit. Just when you're convinced you've won them over and they like you, start being a little less available. And then even less, until they hardly see you at all. You've now effectively instigated the "law of scarcity". We all know this one: people want what they can't have and by constantly being available, you diminish your value. If every time you walked outside your front door there was a huge pile of diamonds to step over, you'd hardly see them as precious would you? The law of scarcity says

> # **The law of scarcity** says don't be at their beck and call. Be around, then **not around** and they'll **fancy you** and like you.

don't be at their beck and call. This will make them fancy you. Be around and then not around and they'll fancy you and like you. I'm stating the obvious here but liking someone is important. We talk loads about chemistry, passion, sexual attraction, and even more about love, yet "like" rarely gets a look in. Opposites don't attract long-term – we search for similarities in a partner. Most of us can't see the point of hanging around friends we don't like, why do it with a lover? Liking someone is more important long-term than actually loving them. It's not just similarities in our personalities that count. Did you know that if you go out with someone who looks like you, they're four times more likely to fall in love with you? "That's so true!", said a girlfriend, when I told her this trivia titbit. "Look at my sister and her husband!" Umm – why? Lisa's sister has bleach-blonde hair, freckles, and ivory skin. Her husband is Indian. "I'm not quite with

you," I said carefully. "I know it's not obvious," she said, "but it's the proportion of their faces. His mother came up to me at their wedding and said 'They will be happy because they are the same. Look at them.'" And it's true. They have the same features, in the same places, in the same proportions."

DON'T DO NICE THINGS FOR THEM, LET THEM DO NICE THINGS FOR YOU

If you do something nice for someone, it makes you feel good on two levels. You feel pleased with yourself and extra-warm towards the person you've just spoilt. To justify the effort or expense, we often over-idealize how wonderful they are to deserve it! End result: we like the person more. When someone does something nice for us, we're pleased. But there are a whole lot of other emotions that come into play – and they're not all good. Sometimes we feel overwhelmed. There's pressure to live up to being the wonderful person who inspired such a gift/act, not to mention pressure to return the favour. It's all even trickier if the "nice thing" comes from someone you quite fancy but aren't sure about yet. Got the point? When we're infatuated with someone, we're desperate to do nice things for them. You're much better off letting them spoil you.

GIVE THEM THE EYE

Harvard psychologist Zick Rubin measured love scientifically by recording the amount of time lovers spent staring at each other. He discovered that couples who are deeply in love, look at each other 75 per cent of the time when talking and are slower to look away when someone dares to intrude. In normal conversation, people look at each other for 30-60 per cent of the time. The significance of what's

now known as Rubin's Scale is obvious: it's possible to tell how "in love" people are by measuring the amount of time they spend gazing adoringly. Some psychologists still use it during counselling to work out how much affection couples feel for each other. It also happens to be remarkably handy information if you want to make someone fall in love with you. Here's how it works: If you look at someone you fancy 75 per cent of the time when they're talking to you, you trick their brain. The brain knows the last time that someone looked at them that long and often, it meant they were in love. So it thinks

---

> PEA is secreted by **the nervous system** when we first fall in love. It makes your palms sweat, **your tummy flip over,** and your heart race.

OK, they're obviously in love with this person as well, and starts to release phenylethylamine (PEA). PEA is a chemical cousin to amphetamines and is secreted by the nervous system when we first fall in love. PEA is what makes your palms sweat, your tummy flip over, and your heart race. The more PEA the person you fancy has pumping through their bloodstream, the more likely they are to fall in love with you. While you can't honestly force someone to adore you if they're not remotely interested, (they won't let you look into their eyes for that long, for a start!) it is entirely possible to kick-start the production of PEA using this technique. Try it. I think you'll be pretty impressed with the results. Give someone the sensation of

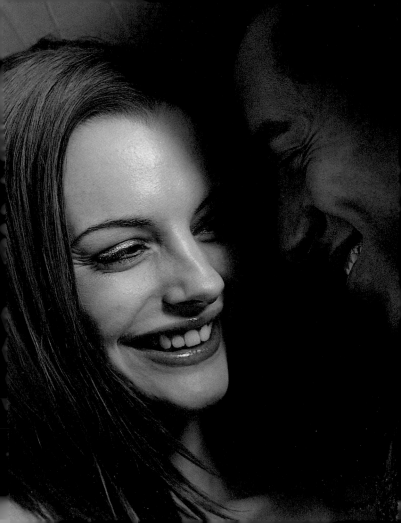

feeling in love whenever they're with you and it's not such a huge leap of logic for them to finally decide that they are!

DON'T LOOK AWAY

There was another crucial finding from Rubin's research: the couples took longer to look away when someone else joined the conversation. Again, if you do this to someone who's not in love with you (yet), you trick their brain into thinking they are and even more PEA floods into their bloodstream. Relationships expert Leil Lownes calls this technique making "toffee eyes". Simply lock eyes with the person you fancy and keep them there, even when they've finished talking or someone else joins the conversation. When you eventually do drag your eyes away (three or four seconds later), do it slowly and reluctantly – as though they're attached by warm toffee. This technique may not sound terribly inspired but, believe me, if done properly it can literally take your breath away. If you're too shy to openly gaze, skip the toffee and think bouncing ball. Look away and at the other person who's joined the conversation, but every time they finish a point or sentence, let your eyes bounce back to the person you fancy. This is a checking gesture – you're checking their reactions to what the speaker is saying – and lets them know you're more interested in them than the other person.

PRACTISE PUPILLOMETRICS

We all know "bedroom eyes" when we see them: it's the look of lust. There's just one thing you need for bedroom eyes: big pupils. According to pupillometrics, the science of pupil study, this is the crucial element we respond to. You can't consciously control your pupils (one reason why people say the eyes don't lie). But you can

create the right conditions to inspire large pupils and get the effect. First, reduce light. Our pupils expand when they're robbed of it, one reason why candlelight and dimmer switches are *de rigueur* in romantic restaurants. It's not just the softening of light that makes our faces appear more attractive, larger pupils also help. Scientists showed two sets of pictures of a woman's face to men. The photograph was identical, except for one thing: the pupils in one set had been doctored to make them larger. When shown the doctored photograph, men judged the woman as twice more attractive than when shown the

> To up the effect of **your bedroom eyes**, focus on the bit of the person you **fancy** the most. (On second thoughts, better make it **the next best thing.**)

real photo. It was repeated with a man's face and tested on women and gave the same result. Our pupils also enlarge when we look at something we like. Again this can be proved using pictures. This time, researchers snuck a picture of a naked woman into a pile of otherwise bland, commonplace photographs then watched men's pupil size when they flicked through. Without exception, the men's pupils expanded on cue. This means if you fancy someone a lot, your pupils are probably already big, black holes. All good. To ensure this is happening or to up the effect of your bedroom eyes, focus on the bit of the person you fancy the most. (On second thoughts, better make it the next best thing.)

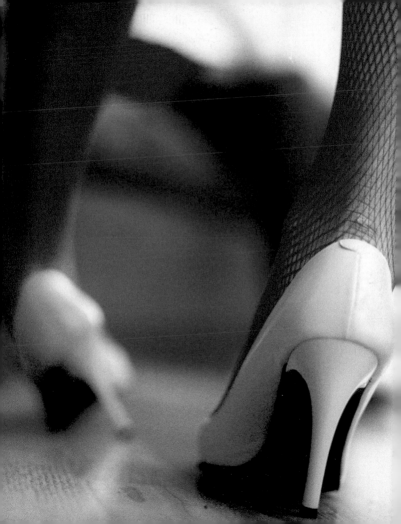

9 Flirting faux pas

Getting sloshed often tops the list for Oh-my-God-I-can't-believe-I-did-that disaster dates. But there are so many less obvious pitfalls...

1. CHIN IN YOUR PALM, ONE ELBOW ON THE TABLE

Not good: The message you're sending when doing this: I'm so bored/tired, I haven't got the energy to hold my head up. It's also a pose we assume when objectively summing someone up since it discourages any physical contact. (You try touching or hugging a friend with one hand stuck under their chin – it feels weird!) Assume this pose after a friend's just told you devastating news and they're likely to be horribly offended (and quite rightly so). If you're not completely confident of your looks, you'll also have a tendency to sit like this. People who like their faces move them around, letting people admire them from all angles (lots of women hold their hair back off their face, to let men have a good look). By looking out from behind your hand, you're hiding most of your face from view. Not a good move. Not even if you're a supermodel.

Try this instead: The only way you can possibly get away with cupping your chin in your palm, is to be truly besotted. Couples in the lovey-dovey honeymoon stage will often simultaneously adopt this posture, slumped on the table, gazing into each other's eyes.

In this situation, the posture switches from showing boredom to adoration. In every other case (excluding 12-year-olds gazing at a popstar poster and those at the beginning of a sexy, sultry love affair) it's to be avoided at all costs. There is no substitute pose – just get those hands away from any type of supportive position.

2. NOT MOVING

Not good: Standing or sitting so still, you look like a rabbit caught in the headlights of an oncoming car.

Try this instead: "People on the move" is a phrase used to describe interesting, dynamic people. Take it as a literal translation. Lots of shy, nervous, insecure people stand very still. Lots of enthusiastic, outgoing, passionate people move around a lot. Note the emphasis on "lots" because this by no means applies to everyone. If you're the type of person who stands so still at a party people start hanging their coats on you, making any sort of movement's got to be a major improvement. By all means practise and perfect all the "good" body language gestures and postures listed in this book but they won't get you anywhere if you simply adopt one position and freeze in it all night. Instead of settling on one way to hold your hands/sit/stand why not master three or four variations? That way you can switch between them all, looking far more relaxed and confident and much less contrived.

3. AWKWARD HANDS

Not good: Wringing your hands, sitting on your hands, balling your hands into tight fists, clutching onto a drink/bag/menu so tightly your fingers go white, fiddling, shredding labels/serviettes – all these signs signal nerves and anxiety. Putting your fingers in your mouth (but not

in a good way) or biting your nails says, "I'm insecure and need reassurance." Sexily sliding a finger suggestively into your mouth is an autoerotic gesture. But there's a huge difference between this and practically shoving your whole hand in there, which is what we tend to do when we're under pressure. Psychologists say it's an unconscious attempt to revert back to the security of breast-feeding:

If you're the type of person who stands so still at a party people starting **hanging coats on you,** making any sort of movement's got to be **a major improvement**

sucking our fingers is the equivalent of sucking on our mother's breast. A bit Freudian I know, but this one actually does make sense. As kids, we replace Mum's breast by sucking on our thumb. Adults often break that habit by biting their nails. (Interesting how most of us bite our thumbnail more than any other.) Theory aside, it looks unattractive. Stop it. Now.

Try this instead: So what should you do with your hands? Shy or nervous people don't move around much, so whatever position they adopt with their hands can look forced. Any position will look awkward if you hold it for too long. The trick is to practise two or three different hand positions in front of a mirror and switch between them. Start by sitting down in front of a table (how you'd usually sit when out to dinner or in a bar), then try the following...

Keep your hands in view: In other words, stop sitting on them or shoving them between your knees. You do it because you don't want people to see they're shaking but people who are lying or hiding something also sit on their hands, so it looks decidedly shifty. Get them up and in view! Rest your forearms on the table, keep your arms open (but not ridiculously wide) and let them drop forwards. They've probably dropped so they're about half a metre apart, your palms are facing towards each other, fingers relaxed but slightly curling inwards. (If your arms are dangling in space, drop them closer to the table. Actually resting on the table is fine.) Now, pretend you're talking to someone (good idea to do these exercises when everyone else is out) and move your hands around, gesturing to back up what you're saying. Continue to use positions where your hands and arms are open and relaxed, your palms rather than the back of your hands are facing the person. It's OK to cross your arms if they're relaxed and loose, if you're leaning forwards with your elbows resting on the table (just don't stay in this position or clutch your arms tightly).

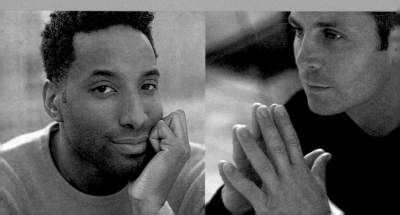

Steepling: A good trick if you're feeling really nervous on a first date is to steeple. Rest your wrists on the table palms facing each other, then spread your hands out, splay your fingers slightly, and press your fingertips together. Touching fingertips has a calming effect and makes you appear more confident. We steeple our hands when we're certain of what we're saying and have no doubt it will be believed: we're in control of a situation. We tend to steeple with fingers pointing upwards while we're talking and downwards while we're listening. Women tend to favour low, unobtrusive steeples, usually pointing down, men tend to steeple higher with fingertips pointing up. In general, the higher the steeple, the more confident you are.

Now stand in front of the mirror and see how your hand gestures translate. The trick is to move them around lots. Wave them about if you feel passionately about something, touch the person you're talking to, preen a little. Do anything other than stand in the classic I'm-terrified position of clutching onto your drink with white knuckles.

We **steeple our hands** when we're **certain** of what we're saying and have no doubt it will be believed: **we're in control** of a situation.

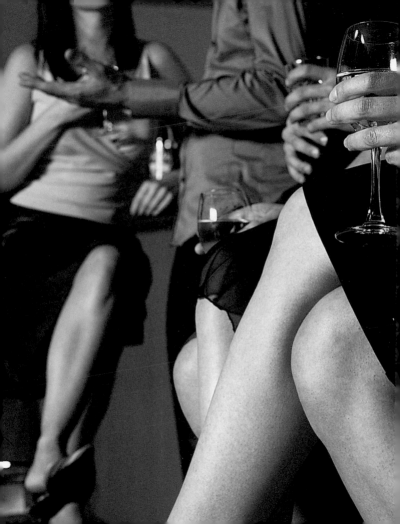

THE ULTIMATE FAUX PAS?

There's nothing worse than misreading the signals and upping the flirting because you think they're interested, only to find out they're so not. Some people send out such clear sexual signals it couldn't be more obvious if they had "You're gorgeous. Want a date?" printed on their t-shirt. With others, it may not be that obvious. Unfortunately, most of us tend to be outstanding flirts and body language decipherers with people we don't particularly fancy and lose the plot entirely when faced with someone we do! So what do you do if you think someone's interested but you're not completely sure? Is there a way to test if they're flirting with you. There certainly is...

Apply the Rule of Four: Don't assume someone's interested in you unless they show a minimum of four separate, positive signals simultaneously and these signals are directed at you. You're looking for what's called "clusters" – lots of body language gestures saying the same thing. The mistake some people make is interpreting body language signals solo. They spot an eyebrow flash and think "Aha! They fancy me." One hour later a foot points towards them and they take that as another sign of interest. Ten minutes on, the person starts preening and they start mentally debating which champagne cocktail to serve at the wedding. Taken separately and aimed generally, body language gestures mean little. Always apply the Rule of Four.

Check your own body language: Are you sending clear signals you're keen on them, such as making eye contact, keeping your body language open and touching them (in a safe place like their arm or shoulder)? Could you be sending out mixed signals? Be honest with yourself. What are your motives for getting together with this person? What are your true feelings? Is your body language leaking what your brain is telling you – you sort of like them but aren't quite sure?

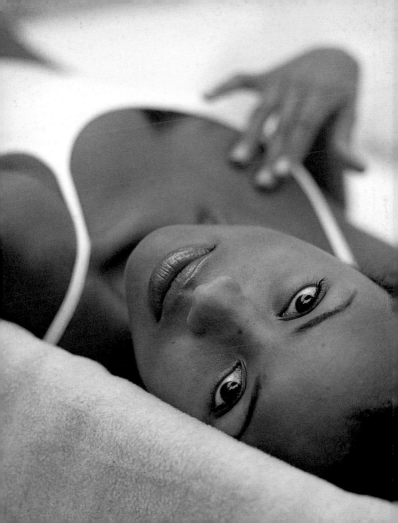

10 Seduction

> So all that flirting's paid off – great! But what do you do when you're face to face with a real-life version of your naughtiest fantasy?

MAKE EVERY MAN WANT YOU...

You've learnt how to package yourself, make an entrance, attract attention, spot who's interested, and respond accordingly...well, now it's Crunch Time. Time to put your money where the pout is. How do you make the transition from full-on-flirt mode to serious seduction? Simple! Read the signs he's ready for more, then watch his body language to ensure you give him exactly what he wants.

SECRET SIGNS HE'S READY FOR SEX...

- He's touching his face more than usual.
- He's holding his head high.
- His eyes appear shiny and moist.
- His pupils are large and dilated.
- His sentences are short and half-finished and he's breathing quickly.
- His thighs tense and his hips start moving in a subtle thrusting motion, suggestive and deliberate.
- His lips are red and swollen.
- His nostrils flare.

GIVE HIM EXACTLY WHAT HE WANTS

- How do you tell if you're really satisfying him? Whatever you do, don't rely on the hardness of his penis! If he's nervous (and who wouldn't be when they finally get to bed a sex goddess like you!), he's focusing way too much on his erection. As a male friend put it so perfectly, erections are like riding a bike: stop and think about it too much and the whole thing goes wobbly. Instead, watch and listen for more reliable signs he's aroused. Is his breathing quick and shallow? Is his skin flushed and pink? Are his lips parted?

- Some guys love women to play innocent in bed, others want their favourite porn film re-enacted. Do both of you a favour by not reading too much into his particular penchant as it's mostly out of his control. Our sexual psyches are programmed from an early age.

- If he's moving closer and pressing hard, he wants it deeper/ harder/a more deliberate touch. If he's pulling away, you're being too rough or fast (or he's losing control and doesn't want to yet).

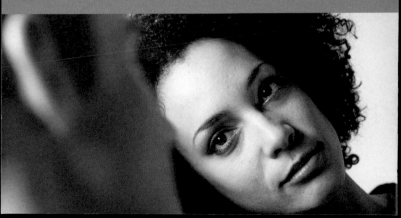

IF YOU REALLY WANT TO MAKE HIS DAY...

- **Be body beautiful** Turn undressing into an art form. Look like you're in your own little world, meanwhile, stay completely body aware so you look gorgeous!
- **Be selfish** Treat him as a tool simply for your pleasure. Straddle him, pull your knickers to one side and use one hand to rub the head of his penis against your clitoris. Have a gloriously self-centred orgasm, then lower yourself onto him during the last stages – not to put him out of his misery but to make your orgasm last longer. (Believe me, he won't complain.)
- **Be bossy** You call the shots and start and stop the action by changing the pace and the place. Jump on top, then off again, then lead him into another room and another position.
- **Be brazen** Most women aren't comfortable being exposed – dare to be different! Show him you're proud of what you've got. Instead of closing your legs when he's admiring the view, spread them wide. The truly secure maintain eye contact too...

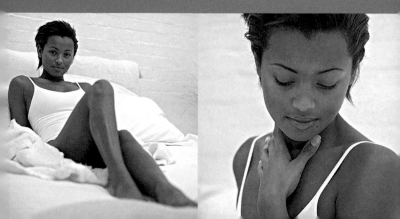

MAKE EVERY WOMAN MELT...

How do you know if a woman wants sex? It'd be a lot easier if your girlfriend was a baboon! Unlike her shy human equivalent, the female baboon blatantly advertizes when she fancies a bit. During ovulation – when she's most likely to get pregnant and feel turned on (also true for humans) – the area round her genitals turns bright red. Just in case her mate doesn't get the message, she crouches in front of him, waving her bottom in the air. While I doubt your girlfriend will wiggle her bottom so blatantly, let's be honest, she is wiggling it. And there are other signs too, albeit a little more subtle.

SECRET SIGNS SHE'S READY FOR SEX...

- Her eyes seem glittery and sparkly.
- Her cheeks change colour, she'll blush and glow, then go pale again. Her pulse is racing.
- Her facial muscles appear tight and toned. Her cheekbones seem more pronounced than usual.

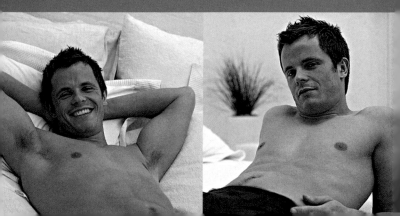

- There's a flush of colour or slight rash on her neck, shoulders, and chest.
- She's stroking her neck lots.
- She's looking at your mouth loads.
- She's touching her mouth and lips with her fingertips.
- She's smoothing her skirt down over her hips to accentuate the curves/tucking her thumbs in the waistband of her trousers/jeans and pushing them down to show off her tummy/hiking her skirt high to show off her thighs.

GIVE HER EXACTLY WHAT SHE WANTS

- Admit it: you love hugging the remote control for the telly. Well, now you're going to do the same with sex. Just as you switch channels to control what's on the screen, you're switching body parts to control the level of her desire. Switching sexual channels not only reduces any chance of desensitization (if touch is constantly concentrated in one area, the skin stops sending

Pull back and **drink in her body** with your eyes, hold **eye contact** during the **naughty bits** – watching each other is an incredible way to **up the eroticism.**

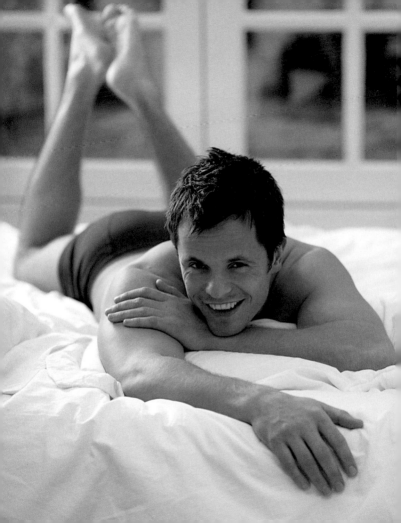

pleasure signals to the brain), it adds an element of surprise and teasing, and keeps her hovering in that almost-but-not-quite-there pre-climax zone. Switch between four basic channels: the visual channel (pull back and drink in her body with your eyes, hold eye contact during naughty bits – watching each other is an incredible way to up the eroticism); the mouth-motivated channel (talking dirty, kissing, biting, licking); the flesh-on-flesh channel (skin-on-skin, touching-at-every-possible-point); the touch channel (gentle fingertip touch, whole-hand massage, grabbing, squeezing, inserting).

- Swap between all four channels to build excitement to a peak, but watch to see which she likes the most. Then settle in to fine-tune your technique. The next session, concentrate on her favourite channel, but continue to throw in plenty of variety and varied techniques until she simply can't choose between them…

IF YOU REALLY WANT TO MAKE HER DAY…

- **Make her beg for it** Push her hand away and say, "You can't touch me until I tell you to." Take off all of her clothes and leave yours on. If you're giving her oral, take regular breaks and detour back up to tongue her belly button, licking your way back down again. Then stop and ask, "How badly do you want me to finish?"
- **Make her cry** – out loud. A lot of women are dreadfully quiet in the bedroom, terrified that even a moan will somehow seem "slutty". (I mean, what would you think? That we're enjoying ourselves? How dreadful!) Give her permission to be vocal by encouraging her to let you know how she's feeling. Ask her to groan when she likes it and keep quiet when she doesn't. Women are natural people pleasers – you'll be the one who's blushing in front of the neighbours.

Sleeping together

It's entirely possible to fake feelings while awake, but you can't fake anything when you're asleep. This is why some experts believe the way you sleep together can reveal lots about your relationship.

LOVING SPOON (TOP LEFT)
The classic "happily married" position: loving but still wanting to be physically close. Few couples hug or spoon during sleep if they're sexually frustrated or resentful. (The partner who's not keen on sex is worried any sign of affection will be interpreted as an invitation).

HONEYMOON (TOP RIGHT)
This is the pose of new lovers smack bang in the honeymoon part of their relationship (the I-can't-believe-I've-found-you bit). It sends three signals: a desire to connect on all levels, a need for reassurance (by hanging on possessively, they can't run away), and total commitment.

BOTTOM TO BOTTOM (BOTTOM LEFT)
It's far more comfortable to sleep solo yet few dispute the joy of sleeping with someone you love. This is a good compromise. Couples who sleep like this are in good shape: it's pretty impressive that you're maintaining contact when unconscious and back to back!

DANGEROUS DISTANCE (BOTTOM RIGHT)
You're back to back at opposite sides of the bed to reduce the chance of touching each other. An arm is 'covering' your heart to protect yourself emotionally. Loads of space between you as you sleep translates to emotional distance during waking hours.

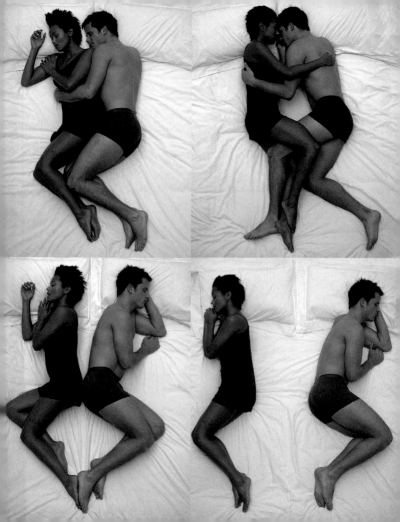

What to say the next day...

Many a great relationship has been halted in full stride by a miserable morning after. Act too keen and you risk being branded as desperate; play it too cool and you risk losing them. The solution? Keep it light and friendly. Here's some solutions to help you make sense of the morning after madness.

I've woken up to find her looking gorgeous, if slightly dishevelled and hung over, in my bed. Every part of me – one in particular – wants to wake her up and do it all over again but I'm scared she'll think all I want her for is sex. Are we supposed to have breakfast first?

Dive straight for the good bits before she's woken up and you'll set the mood for the morning: sexy. If you do really like her make sure it's more soppy-sexy than lusty-sexy because she's likely to be feeling a little vulnerable. Everyone who's got an emotional investment in a relationship feels delicate the day after. You're teenagers again, wondering if they still like you, worrying if you were good enough/too good (aka slutty)/thin/hard/tight enough. Thankfully, there's an instant solution to dissolving these fears: spoon her (see p91, top left). No one spoons comfortably the morning after if they're not interested in at least giving the relationship a try. Connected but facing in the same direction, you don't have to make eye contact (or smell each other's breath) so can wake up, get used to each other, and talk without ever having to meet anyone's eye. Once you've been sufficiently smoochy, make your move sexually. If you feel her body tense with nerves or disapproval, she needs bucketloads of reassurance as well as coffee. Give up, get up, and put the kettle on.

They're leaving early and going straight to work. Where should I say goodbye so that I look interested but not desperate? Is it better to stay in bed or see them to the door?

It depends on the mood, so play it by ear. If they're getting ready in the bedroom and talking to you, it makes sense to stay in bed. It also makes sense to stay put if they don't seem keen. But if they've been cuddly and/or sexy and there's been plenty of "If you knew how hard it is to leave you…" stuff, kiss them goodbye from under the covers, then just as they hit the front door, shout out, "Hold on!" Grab something that barely covers and hold it in front of you as you pad after them in your bare feet. Deliver one final devastatingly sexy snog with your (sort of) naked body pressed firmly against their fully-clothed one, then smile wickedly, stand behind the door, and open it for them to exit. If this doesn't make them come back for more, nothing will.

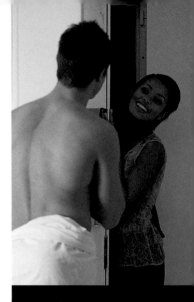

Deliver one final **devastatingly sexy snog** with your (sort of) **naked body pressed** firmly against their fully-clothed one, then **smile wickedly.**

Index

A lot of people stop flirting once they're in a relationship. **Don't.** The couple that plays together **stays together.**

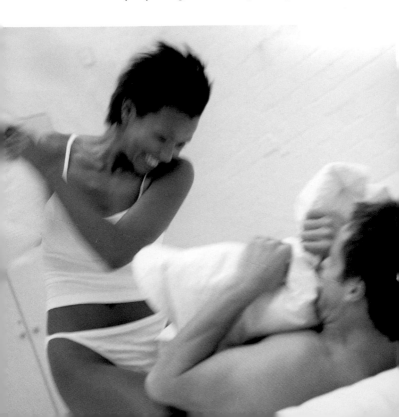

Acknowledgments

The author would like to thank the following people:

First and foremost, thanks to my publishers, DK, who have, as always, treated me like a princess. Thanks go to Corinne Roberts for unwavering and constant support and encouragement along with highly motivational (rather liquid) lunches; ditto my lovely friend Deborah Wright; Christopher Davis for having faith in my projects; Serena Stent and Rachel Kempster for letting the world know about them; and Emma Forge and Carole Ash for doing everything in their power to make the book look great. Enormous thanks especially to my long-suffering editor Peter Jones, who bolstered me up or calmed me down, depending on what was needed, and never once complained while I made a myriad of pointless, miniscule changes which absolutely no-one else would notice except for me.

Nigel and Bev from XAB for once again working their magic to make the book look sensational and Janeanne Gilchrist for the innovative photography.

Vicki McIvor, my much-loved and hard-working agent whose 24/7 professional and emotional support is appreciated far more than she will ever know.

My family who are in my thoughts every second of the day and who I carry with me in my heart wherever I go.

My friends who, once again, not only shared personal anecdotes, read copy, and road-tested techniques but generously forgave me for yet again being unavailable for fun and frolics. Where's the party guys?

At DK
Production Controller: Luca Frassinetti
Production Manager: Lauren Britton
Jacket Editor: Beth Apple
Jacket Designer: Katy Wall

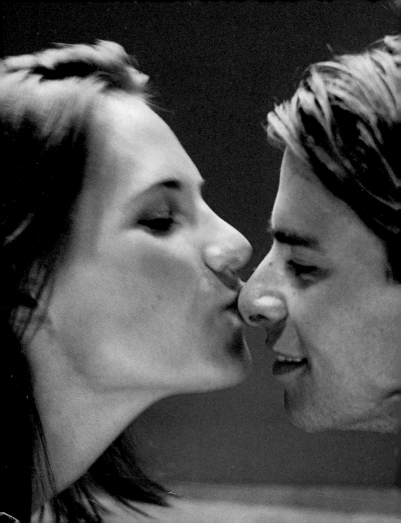